HIV PREVENTION
COMMUNITY
PLANNING GUIDE

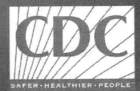

SAFER · HEALTHIER · PEOPLE

I. Introduction

This *Guidance for HIV Prevention Community Planning* defines the Centers for Disease Control and Prevention's (CDC) expectations of health departments and HIV prevention community planning groups (CPGs) in implementing HIV prevention community planning. HIV Prevention Community Planning is one of nine required essential components of a comprehensive HIV prevention program as outlined in *Program Announcement #04012 (2004-2008), HIV Prevention Projects, Notice of Availability of Funds.*

The *HIV Prevention Community Planning Guidance* provides a blue-print for HIV prevention planning and provides flexible direction to CDC grantees* receiving federal HIV prevention funds to design and implement a participatory HIV prevention community planning process. HIV prevention community planning is a collaborative process by which health departments work in partnership with the community to implement a CPG(s) to develop a comprehensive HIV prevention plan that best represents the needs of populations infected with or at risk for HIV.

The Guidance consists of the following sections:

* Section I : Introduction to the Guidance, page 2;
* Section II : Importance of HIV Prevention Community Planning, pages 3-7;
* Section III : HIV Prevention Community Planning Process, pages 8-11
* Section IV : Monitoring and Evaluation, pages 12-14;
* Section V : Roles and Responsibilities, pages 15-20;
* Section VI : Accountability, pages 21-27; and
* Section VII : Appendices, pages 28-46

Note: This current version of the *Guidance for HIV Prevention Community Planning* (text finalized on July 10, 2003) replaces all previous versions and guidances for HIV Prevention Community Planning.

*State/local health departments are the direct grantees of CDC for cooperative agreement HIV prevention funds. Fifty-nine grantees comprised of 50 state health departments; the Washington, D.C. health department; the health departments of Chicago, Houston, Los Angeles, New York City, Philadelphia, and San Francisco; and the health departments of Puerto Rico and the U.S. Virgin Islands are expected to follow this Guidance in implementing HIV prevention community planning.

II. The Importance of HIV Prevention Community Planning

CDC expects HIV prevention community planning to improve HIV prevention programs by strengthening the: (1) scientific basis, (2) community relevance, and (3) population- or risk-based focus of HIV prevention interventions in each project area. Beginning in 1994, CDC changed the manner in which federally-funded state and local level HIV prevention programs were planned and implemented. State, territorial, and local health departments receiving federal prevention funds through CDC were asked to share with representatives of affected communities and other technical experts, the responsibility for developing a comprehensive HIV prevention plan using a process called HIV Prevention Community Planning. The basic intent of the process has been threefold: to increase meaningful community involvement in prevention planning, to improve the scientific basis of program decisions, and to target resources to those communities at highest risk for HIV transmission/acquisition. The CDC remains committed to supporting HIV prevention community planning.

A. CDC HIV PREVENTION STRATEGIC PLAN

HIV Prevention Community Planning plays an important role in achieving the goals of CDC's "HIV Prevention Strategic Plan Through 2005"* (and subsequent strategic plans). CDC's *Overarching National Goal* for HIV prevention in the United States is to:

Reduce the number of new HIV infections in the United States from an estimated 40,000 to 20,000 per year by 2005, focusing particularly on eliminating racial and ethnic disparities in new HIV infections. To accomplish this goal, CDC expects:

---

*Centers for Disease Control and Prevention HIV Prevention Strategic Plan Through 2005. Centers for Disease Control and Prevention, National Center for HIV, STD, and TB Prevention, Atlanta, GA: January 2001 (see CDC's website: http://www.cdc.gov/nchstp/od/hiv_plan/default.htm).

1. By 2005, to decrease by at least 50% the number of persons in the United States at high risk for acquiring or transmitting HIV infection by delivering targeted, sustained, and evidence-based HIV prevention activities.

2. By 2005, through voluntary counseling and testing, increase from the current estimated 70% to 95% the proportion of HIV-infected people in the United States who know they are infected.

3. By 2005, increase from the current estimated 50% to 80% the proportion of HIV-infected people in the United States who are linked to appropriate prevention, care, and treatment services.

4. By 2005, strengthen the capacity nationwide to monitor the epidemic, develop and implement effective HIV prevention interventions, and evaluate prevention programs.

CPGs should be familiar with the CDC Strategic Plan and should work to address the national goal within their jurisdiction's community planning process. However, the local epidemic and needs of the jurisdiction must be a priority for each CPG. Two major components from the strategic plan must be considered by CPGs: (1) targeting populations for which HIV prevention activities will have the greatest impact, and (2) reducing HIV transmission in populations with highest incidence. CPGs must consider the unique issues related to providing HIV prevention for persons living with HIV/AIDS (PLWHA).

B. ADVANCING HIV PREVENTION INITIATIVE

CPGs should also be familiar with CDC's *Advancing HIV Prevention (AHP) Initiative.* Through Advancing HIV Prevention, CDC is refocusing some HIV prevention activities to reduce the number of new HIV infections in the United States.*

Through *Advancing HIV Prevention*, CDC is putting more emphasis on counseling, testing, and referral for the estimated 180,000 to 280,000 persons who are unaware of their HIV infection; partner notification, including partner counseling and referral services; and prevention services for persons living with HIV to help prevent further transmission once they are diagnosed with HIV. In addition, since perinatal HIV transmission can be prevented, CDC is strengthening efforts to promote routine, universal HIV screening as a part of prenatal care. All of this will be accomplished through four strategies: (1) making HIV screening a routine part of medical care; (2) creating new models for diagnosing HIV infection, including the use of rapid testing; (3) improving and expanding prevention services for PLWHA; and, (4) further decreasing perinatal HIV transmission.

Advancing HIV Prevention: New Strategies for a Changing Epidemic — United States, MMWR 2003; 52 (15):329-332.

Advancing HIV Prevention will impact the HIV Prevention Community Planning priority setting process. Because of its potential to substantially reduce HIV incidence, HIV Prevention Community Planning Groups will be required to prioritize HIV-infected persons as the highest priority population for appropriate prevention services. Uninfected, high-risk populations such as sex or needle-using partners of PLWHA, should be prioritized based on local epidemiology and community needs.

C. GOALS OF HIV PREVENTION COMMUNITY PLANNING

The CDC has set three major goals for HIV Prevention Community Planning. The goals provide an overall direction for HIV prevention community planning. In addition, in "Section IV: Monitoring and Evaluation" of the *Guidance*, there are eight objectives that delineate specific processes and products expected for each goal. The three major goals for HIV Prevention Community Planning are:

- GOAL ONE: **Community planning supports broad-based community participation in HIV prevention planning.**

- GOAL TWO: **Community planning identifies priority HIV prevention needs (a set of priority target populations and interventions for each identified target population) in each jurisdiction.**

- GOAL THREE: **Community planning ensures that HIV prevention resources target priority populations and interventions set forth in the comprehensive HIV prevention plan.**

D. GUIDING PRINCIPLES FOR HIV PREVENTION COMMUNITY PLANNING

Guiding Principles for HIV Prevention Community Planning* : To ensure that the HIV prevention community planning process is carried out in a participatory manner, the CDC expects all CPGs to address the following *Guiding Principles of HIV Prevention Community Planning* as they carry out HIV prevention community planning:

1. **The health department and community planning group must work collaboratively to develop a comprehensive HIV prevention plan for the jurisdiction.**

---

*These guiding principles trace their origins to several sources, including various public health planning models; the experience and recommendations of health departments and non-governmental organizations; the health promotion, community development, behavioral and social sciences literature; and CDC and its partners' experience in implementing HIV prevention community planning since 1994.

2. **The community planning process must reflect an open, candid, and participatory process, in which differences in cultural and ethnic background, perspective, and experience are essential and valued.**

3. **The community planning process must involve representatives of populations at greatest risk for HIV infection and PLWHA.** Persons at risk for HIV infection and PLWHA play a key role in identifying prevention needs not adequately met by existing programs and in planning for needed services that are culturally appropriate.

4. **The fundamental tenets of community planning are: parity, inclusion, and representation (often referred to as PIR).** Although these tenets are not accomplished or achieved in a linear fashion, there is a strong relationship between each — with one building on another.

   * *Representation is defined as the act of serving as an official member reflecting the perspective of a specific community.* A representative should truly reflect that community's values, norms, and behaviors (members should have expertise in understanding and addressing the specific HIV prevention needs of the populations they represent). Representatives must be able to participate as group members in objectively weighing the overall priority prevention needs of the jurisdiction.
   * *Inclusion is defined as meaningful involvement of members in the process with an active voice in decision making.* An inclusive process assures that the views, perspectives, and needs of all affected communities are actively included.
   * *Parity is defined as the ability of members to equally participate and carry-out planning tasks/duties.* To achieve parity, representatives should be provided with opportunities for orientation and skills building to participate in the planning process and to have equal voice in voting and other decision-making activities.

5. **An inclusive community planning process includes representatives of varying races and ethnicities, genders, sexual orientations, ages, and other characteristics such as varying educational backgrounds, professions, and expertise.** CPGs should have access to:

   * Persons who reflect the characteristics of the current and projected epidemic in that jurisdiction (as documented by the epidemiologic profile) in terms of age, gender/gender identity, race/ethnicity, sexual orientation, socioeconomic status, geographic and metropolitan statistical area (MSA)-size distribution (urban and rural residence), serostatus, and risk for HIV infection.
   * State and local health department HIV prevention and sexually transmitted disease (STD) treatment staff; staff of state and local education agencies; and staff of other relevant governmental agencies (e.g., substance abuse, mental health, corrections).
   * Experts in epidemiology, behavioral and social sciences, program evaluation, and health planning.
   * Representatives of key non-governmental and governmental organizations providing HIV prevention and related services (e.g., STD, TB, substance abuse prevention and

treatment, mental health services, homeless shelters, prisons/corrections, HIV care and social services, education agencies) to persons with or at risk for HIV infection.

* Representatives of key non-governmental organizations relevant to, but who may not necessarily provide, HIV prevention services (e.g., representatives of business, labor, and faith communities).

6. **The community planning process must actively encourage and seek out community participation.** The community planning process should attempt to accommodate a reasonable number of representatives without becoming so large that it cannot effectively function. Additional avenues for obtaining input on community HIV prevention needs and priorities — especially for input relevant to marginalized populations or to scientific or agency representation that may be difficult to recruit and retain — include:

* Holding well-publicized public meetings,
* Conducting focus groups, and
* Convening ad hoc panels.

7. **Nominations for membership should be solicited through an open process and candidates selection should be based on criteria established by the health department and the community planning group.**

8. **An evidence-based process for setting priorities among target populations should be based on the epidemiologic profile and the community services assessment.**

9. **Priority setting for target populations must address populations for which HIV prevention will have the greatest impact.** Target populations should include populations in which the most HIV infections are occurring or populations with the highest HIV incidence. Moreover, CPGs should discuss the risk behaviors and prevention needs of PLWHA (as PLWHA are included across target populations, their unique needs may not be readily evident) and determine how PLWHA will be included in the priority setting process for target populations.

10. **The set of prevention interventions/activities for prioritized target populations should have the potential to prevent the greatest number of new infections.** CPGs should conceptualize interventions/activities as a set or mix of interventions/activities versus one specific intervention/activity for each target populations.

III. HIV Prevention Community Planning Process

HIV Prevention Community Planning is one of nine required essential components of a comprehensive HIV prevention program. The CDC state/local health department grantee is responsible for carrying out the comprehensive HIV prevention program. As outlined in *Program Announcement #04012 (2004-2008), HIV Prevention Projects, Notice of Availability of Funds*, the nine components are:

1. HIV prevention community planning;
2. HIV prevention activities;
    (a) HIV prevention counseling, testing, and referral services (CTR);
    (b) Partner counseling and referral services (PCRS) with strong linkages to prevention and care services;
    (c) Prevention for HIV-infected persons;
    (d) Health education and risk reduction (HE/RR) activities;
    (e) Public information programs;
    (f) Perinatal Transmission Prevention;
3. Quality assurance;
4. Evaluation of major program activities, interventions, and services, as well as collection of data on interventions and clients served;
5. Capacity-building activities;
6. STD prevention activities;
7. Collaboration and coordination with other related programs;
8. Laboratory support; and,
9. HIV/AIDS epidemiologic and behavioral surveillance.

A. THE COMPREHENSIVE HIV PREVENTION PLAN AND KEY PRODUCTS

The primary task of the CPG is to develop a comprehensive HIV prevention plan that includes prioritized target populations and a set of prevention activities/interventions for each target population. Target populations should be prioritized and prevention activities/interventions chosen based on their ability to prevent as many new infections as possible. Key information necessary to develop the comprehensive HIV prevention plan will be found in the epidemiologic profile and the community services assessment. After developing and/or reviewing these products, CPGs will then move to the task of setting priorities for target populations. Once target populations have been prioritized, the CPG must determine what intervention or mix of interventions will best meet the needs of the prioritized target population. The CPG's comprehensive HIV prevention plan should include details of these key products:

- EPIDEMIOLOGIC PROFILE: describes the impact of the HIV epidemic in the jurisdiction, provides the foundation for prioritizing target populations;

- COMMUNITY SERVICES ASSESSMENT: describes the prevention needs of populations at risk for HIV infection, the prevention activities/interventions implemented to address these needs, and service gaps;

- PRIORITIZED TARGET POPULATIONS: focuses on a set of target populations (identified through the epidemiologic profile and community services assessment) that require prevention efforts due to high rates of HIV infection and high incidence of risky behaviors;

- APPROPRIATE SCIENCE-BASED PREVENTION ACTIVITIES/INTERVENTIONS: a set of prevention activities/interventions (based on intervention effectiveness and cultural/ethnic appropriateness) necessary to reduce transmission in prioritized target populations; and

- LETTER OF CONCURRENCE/CONCURRENCE WITH RESERVATIONS/NON-CONCURRENCE: describes via a written response from the CPG whether the health department application does or does not, and to what degree, agree with the priorities set forth in the Comprehensive HIV Prevention Plan.

The Comprehensive HIV Prevention Plan — **The CPG is required to develop at least one Comprehensive HIV Prevention Plan every five years.** This jurisdiction-wide plan should address all HIV prevention activities and inform decisions about how all HIV prevention funds are to be used, including federal, state, local, and, when possible, private resources. If a jurisdiction implements more than one CPG, the comprehensive plan should summarize any multiple or regional plans into one document. The plan, whether designed to be a one- or multi-year document, must be updated annually. As the health department's federal funding for HIV prevention is on a five-year cycle, the CPG's final plan for the 2004-2008 project period should guide the development of the next five-year funding cycle (January 2009-December 2013).

The CPG should be aware of contracting and funding cycles, and funding sources. Health departments typically implement HIV prevention priorities through a variety of funding mechanisms. Because of multiple-year contracts, shifts in priorities may not affect a program for several years. To understand how resources are being allocated, the CPG should review the health department's most current HIV prevention budget and other sources of prevention funding, and ask the following questions:

- How does it reflect the current priorities?
- What proportion of health department resources have been allocated to these priorities?
- How does the health department distribute resources among prioritized target populations and appropriate science-based prevention activities for each target population?
- What other funding sources — including state, local, and private — were used to address the current priorities?

The Comprehensive HIV Prevention Plan should describe the jurisdiction's entire HIV prevention program. The objective of the plan is to guide how HIV prevention programs in the jurisdiction should respond to the HIV epidemic in implementing HIV prevention community planning, partner counseling and referral services (PCRS), health education/risk reduction (HE/RR), capacity building, evaluation, and other health department activities conducted under *Program Announcement #04012 (2004-2008), HIV Prevention Projects, Notice of Availability of Funds.* The plan must consider all HIV prevention activities regardless of funding. Thus, it is important for the CPG(s) to know and understand the extent and array of prevention funds that will be allocated as a result of both the health department's and other funders' implementation of the CPG's target population priorities and set of prevention activities/intervention, as described in the Comprehensive HIV Prevention Plan.

B. PLANNING CYCLE

The community planning process should be flexible. There is no "one way" to accomplish community planning, however, a process that is based on shared decision making between the health department and the CPG is more likely to accomplish the goals and objectives of community planning. It is important for health departments and CPGs to jointly determine the approach for the community planning cycle (i.e., reasonable time frame and the step-wise process to accomplish the various products of the process that lead to a comprehensive HIV prevention plan and health department application submission requirements).

CPGs should be routinely informed by the health department of other relevant planning efforts. CPGs and health departments should consider merging the HIV prevention community planning process with other planning bodies or processes already in place. In addition to HIV prevention community planning, states and Eligible Metropolitan Areas (EMAs) carry out care planning under the Ryan White Comprehensive AIDS Resources Emergency (CARE) Act. However, if such mergers are undertaken, grantees must adhere to the goals, objectives, principles, and indicators of HIV prevention community planning as described in this *Guidance*.

The health department and CPG are jointly responsible for determining the planning process and cycle and documenting progress made in accomplishing the Goals and Objectives of HIV Prevention Community Planning. To develop a comprehensive HIV prevention plan, a CPG will need access to specific information and products — e.g., epidemiologic profile and community services assessment. Before choosing a timeline for developing a comprehensive plan, it may be important to determine the scope and amount of time that will be necessary to develop and/or review these products, and then to set priorities among target populations and prevention interventions/activities. In determining the planning cycle, health departments and CPGs may choose either one- or multi-year planning processes (from one to five years), and submit a Comprehensive HIV Prevention Plan depending on their planning timeframe. For example:

● **One-Year Process** — if the health department and the CPG decide to complete the planning process in one year, then all of the products of community planning and the comprehensive HIV prevention plan must be completed in time for the annual health department application process.

● **Two-Year Process** — if the health department and the CPG decide to complete the planning process in two years, then all of the products of community planning and the comprehensive HIV prevention plan must be completed within two years. In year one, the CPG is required to update the most recent comprehensive HIV prevention plan and carry-out a concurrence process. In the second year, the CPG is required to develop a new comprehensive HIV prevention plan and carry out a concurrence process.

● **Multiple-Year Process** *(three to five years)* — if the health department and the CPG decide to complete the planning process over multiple years, then all of the products of community planning and the comprehensive HIV prevention plan must be completed within either three, four, or five years. Each year, the CPG is required, depending on the time frame chosen, to either update the most recent comprehensive HIV prevention plan and carry-out a concurrence process or to develop a new comprehensive HIV prevention plan and carry out a concurrence process.

Note: Regardless of the planning timeframe, due to potential changes in funding, each year the CPG is required to either update the most recent comprehensive HIV prevention plan and carry-out a concurrence process or to develop a new comprehensive HIV prevention plan and carry out a concurrence process.

IV. Monitoring and Evaluation of HIV Prevention Community Planning

The monitoring and evaluation of HIV prevention community planning is based on the three goals and eight objectives for HIV Prevention Community Planning. Each goal provides an overall direction for community planning. The goals are broad, however, the objectives delineate specific processes and products expected for each goal. In addition, fifty-two critical attributes have been designated to monitor implementation of each objective (see **Appendix C** for a complete list of attributes; note: jurisdictions are not required to individually report on each attribute listed). For example, if the designated attributes of an objective for a given jurisdiction are present in a community planning process, then there is an indication that the objective is being met.

Required activities to monitor and evaluate the extent to which each HIV prevention community planning goal and objective is being met is described in the most current CDC Evaluation *Guidance*. The *Evaluation Guidance* provides details on: (1) conducting an annual CPG membership survey, (2) describing priority populations, (3) describing their accompanying set of prevention/ interventions activities, and (4) assessing the linkages between the comprehensive HIV prevention plan and the CDC funding application, as well as the linkages between the plan and the funded interventions. Furthermore, four program performance indicators have been developed for HIV prevention community planning (see "Section VI: Accountability"). These indicators allow jurisdictions to obtain a snapshot of HIV prevention community planning implementation and provide findings to make improvements in the planning process. Data sources for these indicators are based on monitoring and evaluation activities in the *Evaluation Guidance*.

Monitoring and evaluation of HIV Prevention Community Planning is a shared responsibility between the health department and the CPG. However, health departments have the ultimate responsibility in reporting their monitoring and evaluation activities to CDC as required by

Program Announcement 04012 and the Evaluation Guidance. The CDC is responsible for providing leadership in the evaluation of HIV prevention community planning, and the provision of evaluation technical assistance to effectively evaluate the community planning process.

The following Goals and Objectives of HIV prevention community planning provide a framework for monitoring and measuring progress in achieving a reduction of new HIV infections and reduced HIV-related morbidity.

GOAL ONE — **Community planning supports broad-based community participation in HIV prevention planning.**

The Objectives that will be monitored and measured to determine progress in achieving Goal One:

- *Objective A: Implement an open recruitment process (outreach, nominations, and selection) for CPG membership.*

- *Objective B: Ensure that the CPG(s) membership is representative of the diversity of populations most at risk for HIV infection and community characteristics in the jurisdiction, and includes key professional expertise and representation from key governmental and non-governmental agencies.*

- *Objective C: Foster a community planning process that encourages inclusion and parity among community planning members.*

GOAL TWO — **Community planning identifies priority HIV prevention needs (a set of priority target populations and interventions for each identified target population) in each jurisdiction.**

The Objectives that will be monitored and measured to determine progress in achieving Goal Two:

- *Objective D: Carry out a logical, evidence-based process to determine the highest priority, population-specific prevention needs in the jurisdiction.*

- *Objective E: Ensure that prioritized target populations are based on an epidemiologic profile and a community services assessment.*

- *Objective F: Ensure that prevention activities/interventions for identified priority target populations are based on behavioral and social science, outcome effectiveness, and/or have been adequately tested with intended target populations for cultural appropriateness, relevance, and acceptability.*

GOAL THREE— **Community planning ensures that HIV prevention resources target priority populations and interventions set forth in the comprehensive HIV prevention plan.**

The Objectives that will be monitored and measured to determine progress in achieving Goal Three:

- *Objective G: Demonstrate a direct relationship between the Comprehensive HIV Prevention Plan and the Health Department Application for federal HIV prevention funding.*

- *Objective H: Demonstrate a direct relationship between the Comprehensive HIV Prevention Plan and funded interventions.*

V. Roles and Responsibilities

Each member of the CPG has a specific role to play whether reflecting the perspective of a specific community, co-chairing, leading a committee or work group, or staffing the community planning process. There are specific roles and responsibilities that the **health department** and **CPG** are each expected to perform in implementing the community planning process. In addition, there are **shared responsibilities** between the health department and the CPG, and specific roles and responsibilities related to CDC's support and monitoring of HIV prevention community planning.

> HEALTH DEPARTMENTS — Health Departments are responsible for supporting the HIV prevention community planning process (via funding, staff and/or consultant/contractor resources, and leadership). The Health Department's role in HIV prevention community planning is to:

1. **Create and maintain at least one CPG that meets the goals and objectives and operating principles described in this** *Guidance*.
   * If there is more than one CPG in the jurisdiction, the health department is responsible for deciding how best to integrate statewide, regional, and local community planning.
   * If there are multiple jurisdictions within a state (i.e., Los Angeles, San Francisco, and California; Chicago and Illinois; Philadelphia and Pennsylvania; New York City and New York; and Houston and Texas), the state and local jurisdictions are expected to have ready access to and review each other's comprehensive HIV prevention plans.

   In addition, it is the health department's responsibility to support community planning activities, including:
   * Supporting meeting logistics (CPG, public, and other input-focused meetings).
   * Supporting CPG member involvement (such as transportation, expense reimbursement, etc.), especially for persons with or at risk for HIV infection.
   * Supporting infrastructure for the HIV prevention community planning process (such as staff, consultants, contracts, etc.).

2. **Appoint the Health Department Co-Chair.** If a state health department implements multiple CPGs, they may encourage local health departments to serve as the Health Department Co-Chair of such planning groups.

3. **Ensure collaboration between community planning and other relevant planning processes in the jurisdiction** such as Ryan White CARE Act planning (Titles I, II, III, and IV) and STD prevention.

4. **Develop the epidemiologic profile and conduct the community services assessment.** Because the health department has a responsibility to inform the public about emerging public health trends, including HIV/AIDS and other related health issues such as syphilis among MSM, it is responsible for developing both of these products (which may be developed by the health department or via a consultant or contract). However, the health department should discuss each of the products with the CPG and agree on the approach that will be used to develop the epidemiologic profile (e.g., types of data desired, format, etc.) and the community services assessment (e.g., types of data to be collected, the methodologies to be used, format, etc.).

5. **Provide the CPG with information on other federal/state/local public health services for high-risk populations identified in the comprehensive HIV prevention plan.**
   * For example, STD prevention and treatment, TB, hepatitis services, etc.

6. **Assure that CPGs have access to current information (including relevant budget information) related to HIV prevention and analysis of the information, including potential implications for HIV prevention in the jurisdiction.** Sources of information include evaluations of program activities, local program experience, programmatic research, the best available science, and other sources, especially as it relates to the at-risk population groups within a given community and the priority needs identified in the comprehensive plan.

7. **Develop an application to the CDC for federal HIV prevention cooperative agreement funds based on the comprehensive HIV prevention plan(s) developed through the HIV prevention community planning process.**
   * Allocate resources based on the priorities presented in the comprehensive HIV prevention plan.
   * Present the funding application and budget to the CPG with adequate time for the CPG to review and issue a written response.
   * Demonstrate that the community planning process has met the Goals and Objectives of community planning.

8. **Allocate, administer and coordinate public funds (including state, federal, and local) to prevent HIV transmission and reduce HIV-associated morbidity and mortality.**
   * Award HIV prevention funds to implement the HIV prevention services stated in the comprehensive HIV prevention plan and health department application.
   * Monitor contractor (service provider) activities and document contractor compliance.

9. **Provide regular updates to the CPG on successes and barriers encountered in implementing the HIV prevention services described in the comprehensive HIV prevention plan.**
   * Provide the CPG with local program evaluation data, where available.

10. **Report progress and accomplishments to CDC.**

HIV PREVENTION COMMUNITY PLANNING GROUPS — CPGs are responsible for developing a comprehensive HIV prevention plan and reviewing the health department's application for federal HIV prevention funding for concurrence with the plan. CPGs do not allocate resources.

The CPG's role in HIV prevention community planning is to:

---

1. **Elect the Community Co-Chair(s), who will work with the health department-designated co-chair(s).**

2. **Review and use key data to establish prevention priorities.** The CPG should review all existing and new products (i.e., epidemiologic profile, community services assessment, prioritized target populations, selected set of prevention activities/interventions, and the comprehensive HIV prevention plan) prior to all decision making.

3. **Develop a Comprehensive HIV Prevention Plan.**
   * The CPG's emphasis should be on developing a comprehensive HIV prevention plan that includes priority target populations and prevention activities/interventions. Target populations should be prioritized and prevention activities/interventions chosen based on their ability to prevent as many new infections as possible.
   * The health department and CPG, together, determine if the CPG will take on responsibility for more than planning-related activities.

4. **Collaborate with the health department in reviewing and finalizing key community planning activities:** the epidemiologic profile, the community services assessment, prioritized target populations, set of prevention activities/interventions, and the comprehensive plan for HIV prevention community planning.

5. **Review the health department application to CDC for federal HIV prevention funds, including the proposed budget, and develop a written response that describes whether the health department application does or does not, and to what degree, agree with the priorities set forth in the comprehensive HIV prevention plan.**
   * This is often called the concurrence/non-concurrence process.

1. **Process Management:** Develop procedures/policies* that address membership, roles, and decision making, specifically:
   * Composition of the CPG; selection, appointment, and duration of terms to ensure that the CPG membership reflects, as much as possible, the epidemic in the jurisdiction (i.e., age, race/ethnicity, gender, sexual orientation, geographic distribution, and risk for HIV infection);
   * Roles and responsibilities of the CPG, its members, and its various components (i.e., committees, work groups, regional groups, etc.);
   * Process to prospectively identify potential conflict(s) of interest and methods for resolution of conflict(s) of interest for CPG members.
   * Methods for reaching decisions; attendance at meetings; and resolution of disputes identified in planning deliberations.

2. **Membership Selection:** Develop and apply criteria for selecting CPG members:
   * Special emphasis should be placed on procedures for identifying representatives of at-risk, affected, and socioeconomically marginalized groups that are underserved by existing HIV prevention programs.

3. **Input Mechanisms:** Determine the most effective input mechanisms for the community planning process.
   * The process must be structured to best incorporate and address needs and priorities identified at the community level.
   * The process should include strategies for obtaining input from key populations (e.g., IDUs, MSM, youth, undocumented immigrants, etc.) that may not be CPG members.

4. **Planning Funds**: Provide input on the use of planning funds:
   * Support CPG meetings, public meetings, and other means for obtaining community input;
   * Facilitate involvement of all participants in the planning process, particularly those persons with and at risk for HIV infection;
   * Support capacity development for inclusion, representation, and parity of community representatives and for other CPG members to participate effectively in the process;
   * Provide technical assistance to health departments and community planning groups by outside experts;
   * Assure representation of the CPG (governmental and non-governmental) at necessary regional or national planning meetings;
   * Support planning infrastructure for the HIV prevention community planning process;
   * Collect, analyze, and disseminate relevant data; and
   * Monitor and evaluate the community planning process.

---

*All procedures/policies should be consistent with the Guiding Principles of HIV prevention community planning (Section II of this *Guidance*) and developed with input from both the CPG and the health department.

5. **Provide a thorough orientation for all new members, as soon as possible after appointment.** New members should understand the:
   * Goals and Core Objectives, roles, responsibilities, and principles outlined in this *Guidance*;
   * Procedures and ground rules used in all deliberations and decision making; and
   * Specific policies and procedures for resolving disputes and avoiding conflicts of interest that are consistent with the principles of this *Guidance*.

6. **Evaluate the community planning process to assure that it is meeting the core objectives of community planning.**

CENTERS FOR DISEASE CONTROL AND PREVENTION — The role of the CDC in the HIV Prevention Community Planning process is to:

---

1. **Provide leadership in the national design, implementation, and evaluation of HIV prevention community planning.**

2. **Collaborate with health departments, CPGs, national organizations, federal agencies, and academic institutions to ensure the provision of technical/program assistance and training for the community planning process.**
   * Work with the health department and the community co-chairs to provide technical/program assistance for the community planning process, including discussing roles and responsibilities of community planning participants, disseminating CDC documents, and responding to direct inquiries to ensure consistent interpretation of the guidance.

3. **Provide technical/program assistance through a variety of mechanisms to help recipients understand how to:**
   * Analyze epidemiologic, behavioral, and other relevant data to assess the impact and extent of the HIV/AIDS epidemic in defined populations;
   * Analyze community services assessments and compile analyses of prevention program gaps;
   * Prioritize target populations, and interventions based on their ability to result in the greatest decrease in new HIV infections;
   * Identify and evaluate effective and cost-effective HIV prevention activities for these priority populations;
   * Provide access to needed behavioral and social science expertise;
   * Ensure PIR in the community planning process;
   * Identify and manage dispute and conflict of interest issues; and
   * Evaluate the community planning process.

4. **Alert health departments and CPGs about emerging trends or changes in the HIV/AIDS epidemic.**

5. **Provide leadership in the coordination between health departments, CPGs, directly-funded community-based organizations (CBOs).** CDC will provide leadership for internal collaboration that may impact HIV prevention programs and funding.

6. **Monitor the HIV prevention community planning process for implementation of the three goals and eight objectives.**

7. **Collaborate with health departments in evaluating HIV prevention programs.**

8. **Collaborate with other federal agencies and offices** (particularly the Health Resources and Services Administration, National Institutes of Health, Office of HIV/AIDS Policy, Office on Minority Health, and the Substance Abuse and Mental Health Services Administration) in promoting the transfer of new information and emerging prevention technologies or approaches (i.e., epidemiologic, biomedical, operational, behavioral, or evaluative) to health departments and other prevention partners, including non-governmental organizations.

VI. Accountability

CDC Expectations – CDC is committed to the concept of HIV prevention community planning as outlined in this *Guidance*. CDC will monitor the progress health departments and CPGs are making in meeting these expectations through a select number of required indicators. In summary, CDC expects that:

- Health departments will support a collaborative community planning process, including providing sufficient financial resources, in compliance with the eight objectives and guiding principles;

- Priority target populations and a recommended set of interventions/activities identified in the comprehensive HIV prevention plan are based on: (a) having the greatest impact on reducing HIV transmission, and (b) reducing HIV transmission in populations with highest incidence. Priority target populations and prevention interventions/activities should be consistent with the epidemiologic profile, community services assessment, and behavioral/social science data presented in the plan;

- CPGs will review the entire health department application for federal HIV prevention funds, including the budget, prior to writing letters of concurrence, concurrence with reservations or nonconcurrence; and

- The allocation of CDC-awarded resources should be consistent with the prioritized target populations and set of appropriate prevention interventions/activities as described in the comprehensive HIV prevention plan.

A. PROGRAM PERFORMANCE INDICATORS

Program Performance Indicators — The following required indicators provide a gauge for HIV prevention community planning implementation specifically in processes, activities, and/or products that must be developed or implemented to achieve the goals and objectives of HIV prevention community planning. The data sources detail what data will be reported to CDC.

Furthermore, CDC will provide specific guidance on how performance indicators will be operationalized and reported and also how to set baselines and targets for each indicator.

• **Indicator E.1: Proportion of populations most at risk, as documented in the epidemiologic profile, that have at least one CPG member that reflects the perspective of each population**

National Data Source:		PEMS: Community Planning Membership Survey, The Epidemiologic Profile
Measure:	*Numerator:*	The number of populations most at risk (as documented in the epidemiologic profile that have at least one CPG member that reflects the perspective of each population.
	Denominator:	Number of populations most at risk (up to 10) as documented in the epidemiologic profile.

Measure(s) Used to Obtain the Data: Epidemiological Profile CPG Membership Survey

---

• **Indicator E.2: Proportion of key attributes of an HIV prevention community planning process that CPG membership agreed have occurred.**

National Data Source:		PEMS: Community Planning Membership Survey
Measure:	*Numerator:*	The total number of key attributes of which CPG members agreed occurred.
	Denominator:	The total number of valid responses ("agree" or "disagree").

Measure(s) Used to Obtain the Data: HIV Prevention Community Planning Membership Survey

---

• **Indicator E.3: Percent of prevention interventions/supporting activities in the health department CDC funding application specified as a priority in the comprehensive HIV prevention plan.**

National Data Source:		PEMS: Community Planning Linkage Table Worksheet
Measure:	*Numerator:*	The number of prevention/ other supporting activities in the health department CDC funding application specified as a priority in the comprehensive HIV prevention plan.
	Denominator:	The number of all prevention/ other supporting activities identified in the health department CDC funding application.

Measure(s) Used to Obtain the Data: Community Planning Linkage Table Worksheet

---

* **Indicator E.4: Percent of health department-funded prevention interventions/supporting activities that correspond to priorities specified in the comprehensive HIV prevention plan.**

> *National Data Source:* PEMS: Community Planning Linkage Table Worksheet & Process Monitoring System
>
> *Measure:* **Numerator:** The number of funded prevention/ other supporting activities that correspond to priorities specified in the most current comprehensive HIV prevention plan.
>
> *Denominator:* The number of all funded prevention/ other supporting activities.
>
> *Measure(s) Used to Obtain the Data:* Community Planning Linkage Table Worksheet, Program Monitoring and Evaluation System

Note: For more guidance or information on these HIV Prevention Community Planning indicators, please reference CDC's *Technical Assistance Guidelines for Health Department HIV Prevention Program Performance Indicators.*

B. CONCURRENCE, CONCURRENCE WITH RESERVATIONS OR NONCONCURRENCE

Letter of Concurrence, Concurrence with Reservations, or Nonconcurrence — As part of its application to the CDC for federal HIV prevention funds, every health department must include a letter of concurrence or nonconcurrence from each CPG officially convened and recognized in the jurisdiction.

CPG members should carefully review the comprehensive HIV prevention plan and the health department's entire application (including the proposed budget) to CDC for federal funds.
* It is the responsibility of the health department to provide the CPG with ample time to review the health department's application.
* Health departments should provide the CPG with the jurisdiction's "Community Planning Linkage Table Worksheet" showing how the priorities identified in the plan are being addressed in the jurisdiction and which priorities specifically are being addressed in the application for CDC funding.
* It is the responsibility of the CPG to determine whether the health department's application reflects the priorities of the CPG's comprehensive HIV prevention plan.

It is critical that the CPG review the proposed allocation of resources in the health department's application using the "Community Planning Linkage Table Worksheet." In reviewing the application, CPGs are reminded that:
* CPGs are not asked to review and comment on internal health department issues such as salaries of individual health department staff or funding to specific HIV prevention services agencies,

- The letter of concurrence or nonconcurrence directly relates to the jurisdiction's proposed allocation of CDC funds for HIV prevention, and
- The community planning process requires setting priorities for target populations and a recommended mix of prevention interventions for each population.

Letters of concurrence, concurrence with reservations, nonconcurrence should indicate:

☐ That the CPG was provided with a copy of the comprehensive HIV prevention plan and the health department's application for federal HIV funding, including the budget;

☐ The degree to which ("how well or not") the health department and CPG has successfully collaborated in developing, reviewing, or revising the comprehensive HIV prevention plan;

☐ The degree to which the health department has responded to the priorities in the comprehensive HIV prevention plan in its application to the CDC for federal HIV prevention funds;

☐ The process used for obtaining concurrence, including:
  - A description of the process used by the CPG to review the application;
  - The amount of time the CPG had to review the application;
  - Who from the CPG reviewed the application (e.g., co-chairs, members, subcommittee chairs, etc.);
  - The degree of concurrence (i.e., without reservation, with reservations, or non-concurrence); and

☐ At a *minimum*, the letter(s) should be signed by the co-chairs of each CPG on behalf of the CPG. The letter should include an indication that the Co-Chairs have reviewed and understand the application, are signing the letter on behalf of the CPG, and will report on the concurrence process to the entire CPG.

The Letter of **concurrence** may include **reservations** or a statement of concern/issues. The health department will be required to address these reservations or concerns in an addendum to the HIV prevention application.

Letter(s) of **nonconcurrence** indicate that the HIV prevention community planning group disagrees with the program priorities identified in the health department's application. The letter should cite specific reasons for nonconcurrence. In instances when a health department does not concur with the recommendations of the HIV prevention community planning group(s) and believes that public health would be better served by funding HIV prevention activities/services that are substantially different, the health department must submit a letter of explanation in its application. **CDC will assess and evaluate these explanations on a case-by-case basis and determine what action may be appropriate.**

When CDC receives a letter of nonconcurrence or if the health department does not meet the requirements specified by this *Guidance*, actions may include any of the following:

- Obtaining more input/information regarding the situation;
- Meeting with the health department and co-chairs;
- Negotiating with the health department regarding the issues raised;
- Recommending local mediation;
- Requesting that the health department provide a detailed corrective action plan to address areas of concern and specify a timeframe for completion;
- Conducting an on-site comprehensive program assessment to identify and propose action steps to resolve areas of concern;
- Conducting an on site program assessment focused on a specific area(s);
- Developing a detailed technical assistance plan for the project area to help systematically address the situation;
- Placing conditions or restrictions on the award of funds pending a future submission by the applicant; and
- Loss of funding in future applications, if nonconcurrence or poor performance is not satisfactorily addressed.

In the event of the availability of supplemental funds for HIV prevention, CDC will require a letter of concurrence for health department applications for such funds. A Letter of Concurrence for Supplemental Funds will be expected to address the criteria above.

Sample letters of concurrence, concurrence with reservations or nonconcurrence are included in **Appendix B.**

VII. Appendices

A. Conflict of Interest

B. Sample Letters of Concurrence, Concurrence with Reservations or Nonconcurrence

C. Critical HIV Prevention Community Planning Attributes

D. Glossary of HIV Prevention Terms

APPENDIX A: Conflict of Interest

CONFLICT OF INTEREST

While the *American Heritage Dictionary of the English Language* defines conflict of interest simply as "conflict between the private interests and the public obligations of a person in an official position," your CPG may wish to provide a more precise definition.

Conflict of interest occurs when:

1. An appointed voting member of the CPG has a direct fiduciary interest (which includes ownership; employment; contractual; creditor, or consultative relationship to; or Board or staff membership) in an organization (including any such interest that existed at any time during the twelve months preceding her/his appointment), with which the CPG has a direct, financial and/or recognized relationship; and/or

2. When a member of the CPG knowingly takes action or makes a statement intended to influence the conduct of the CPG in such a way as to confer any financial benefit on the member, family member(s), or on any organization in which s/he is an employee or has a significant interest."

REVIEW OR DEVELOP CONFLICT OF INTEREST STATEMENTS

Conflicts of interest often occur when CPG members who are advocates for particular groups take part in a process intended to meet the needs of many groups. For example, the executive director of a homeless youth organization is likely to push issues affecting homeless youth. While that is understandable (and even desirable in many cases), a CPG requires an objective process based on data. Your CPG members must consider how priority setting will affect all populations being considered. Although the executive director's job depends on a commitment to the interests of homeless youth, this member must base his/her decisions on the epidemiologic profile and other data characterizing the jurisdiction's HIV epidemic.

Conflicts of interest must not rule the group. They are not inherently bad, but if your group doesn't deal with these openly, they may bias your process. To ensure a fair outcome, your group can take certain key steps to lessen the conflict of interest problem.

Your CPG already may have established some policies and mechanisms for addressing conflicts of interest. If so, refer to those before beginning the priority setting process. If your CPG has not developed such policies, you should do so before beginning the priority setting process. The policies take time to develop, but these will save much time later by limiting conflicts of interest.

State and local laws often define conflict of interest. Contact your county or state attorney general's office for a specific legal definition.

By reviewing or developing your CPG's conflict of interest policies, your group can assure a fair process that includes diverse participants.

Key Steps to Avoid Conflicts of Interest

☐ Develop a definition of conflict of interest that all members accept and agree to abide by.

☐ Develop a policy stating how the CPG will deal with apparent conflicts of interest. This policy varies greatly from group to group. It includes everything from barring participation in any discussion and voting related to the conflict to allowing participation in the discussions but not in the voting. The key is agreeing upon a procedure for addressing conflicts of interest before any conflicts — real or perceived — arise.

☐ Create a process that enables all community planning members to disclose conflicts of interest to the CPG. It helps to have a process that includes a written form and to keep these forms accessible to all members. It also helps to have a specific group, committee, or individual be responsible for oversight of the disclosure process.

☐ Clarify in writing the consequences of not cooperating with the conflict of interest policy. CPG members should be fully aware of the gravity of violating the policy.

APPENDIX B: Sample Letters of Concurrence, Concurrence with Reservations or Nonconcurrence

SAMPLE 1 - Statewide Community Planning Group: *LETTER OF CONCURRENCE*

Date

Mr./Ms._____

Grants Management Officer

Procurement and Grants Office

Centers for Disease Control and Prevention

290 Brandywine Road

Room 300, Mailstop E-15

Atlanta, GA 30341

Dear Mr./Ms._____:

The_____HIV community planning group confirmed by consensus at its meeting August 8-9, 2003, its concurrence with the state of _____'s application to CDC for HIV prevention funds under program announcement 04012. The planning group has reviewed the state's proposed 2004 objectives, activities, and budget and finds them to be responsive to the priorities identified by the planning group and expressed in the _____ HIV prevention plan, 2003-2005.

The planning group met _____ (frequency) during 2003 and through a series of full-group and subcommittee meetings planned the content of meetings, defined needs established in the existing plan, and developed a schedule to review the state's HIV prevention application. Members were asked to review materials (the HIV prevention plan 2003-2005 and the state's 2004 AIDS/STD program plan objectives) and be prepared to discuss them at the September meeting. Thirteen of the 16 planning group members reviewed progress on the state's 2003 objectives, the planning group priorities, the HIV prevention plan 2003-2005, and the state's draft 2004 program plan and objectives. At the August planning group meeting, members gave AIDS/STD program staff considerable feedback on content for the 2004 CDC application. Based on a review of the draft program plan, the planning group easily reached consensus on its concurrence that the priorities and strategies proposed for the state's application reflected the priorities expressed in the planning group's plan.

The two community co-chairs, along with the health department co-chair, have been designated as signatories to the letter of concurrence.

Sincerely,

SAMPLE 2 - Statewide Community Planning Group, with Regional Community Planning Groups:
LETTER OF CONCURRENCE

Date
Mr./Ms._____
Grants Management Officer
Procurement and Grants Office
Centers for Disease Control and Prevention
290 Brandywine Road
Room 300, Mailstop E-15
Atlanta, GA 30341

Dear Mr./Ms. _____:

On behalf of the statewide HIV/STD community planning group (CPG), we are confirming our concurrence with the 2004 _____ prevention plan and grant application. We believe that these documents address the prevention needs of priority populations and are being supported through the funding commitments of the health department. We feel strongly that the 2005 Plan and grant application reflect the planning efforts of the statewide HIV/STD community planning group and that a thorough review process was used to ensure concurrence. Our process included:

* The statewide resources development committee reviewed the proposed budget for 2005 at the June 2004 statewide meeting. All members of the statewide CPG received time to provide input (until early June). No one voiced opposition to the committee.
* A presentation of all regional plans to the statewide CPG ensured that the statewide CPG was aware of regional priorities. A review team composed of the statewide community co-chair, regional representatives, at-large members, and gallery participants read the plan and the regional plans to ensure that the state plan was based on the regional plans.
* A second-review team composed of the statewide community co-chair, a new set of regional representatives, at-large members, and gallery participants, read the application and reviewed regional plans to ensure that the application met CDC guidelines.
* At the September meeting of the Statewide CPG, the Resource Development Committee presented the budget, reporting that the budget adequately reflected the priorities presented in the comprehensive plan. The plan review team followed the same process. The statewide CPG voted to accept the plan. The grant application review team followed the same process, and the CPG voted to accept the application.

We look forward to implementing the plan to reduce the spread of HIV in _____.

Sincerely,

State Health Department Co-Chair State Community Co-Chair
Region X Co-Chairs, Region X Co-Chairs
Region X Co-Chairs, Region X Co-Chairs

SAMPLE 3 - Statewide Community Planning Group:
LETTER OF CONCURRENCE WITH RESERVATIONS

Date
Grant Management Officer
Grants Management Branch
Procurement and Grants Office
Centers for Disease Control and Prevention
290 Brandywine Road
Room 300, Mailstop E-15
Atlanta, GA 30341
Re: LETTER OF CONCURRENCE WITH RESERVATIONS

Dear Mr./Ms._____:

We concur with our health department's application with one major exception. We are concurring with concerns to the health department's application for funding. As a CPG, we feel that the health department has consistently failed to implement effective programs for Men who Have Sex with Men (MSM). We recognize that this is a difficult population to reach, however, this is the jurisdictions's number one target population (as documented in both the epidemiologic profile and our priority setting process). The CPG has stated both the need and the types of interventions that are most needed (see the Comprehensive HIV Prevention Plan, Target Populations: MSM).

Despite our reservations about the application, we feel proud of how the _____ community planning group came together with the health department and accomplished so much with such a diverse group of individuals. The_____ community planning process is truly community driven. This was reflected in the review of the health department's application. The health department distributed copies of the application to all members and each member had ten days to review the application and to respond with comments. The community co-chairs collated comments and then participated in a conference call to make the decision to concur with concerns with the health department application.

We remain united in the struggle for healthy communities!

The _____ Community Planning Group

SAMPLE 4 - Statewide Community Planning Group:
LETTER OF NONCONCURRENCE

Date
Grants Management Officer
Procurement and Grants Office
Centers for Disease Control and Prevention
290 Brandywine Road
Room 300, Mailstop E-15
Atlanta, GA 30341
Re: LETTER OF NONCONCURRENCE

Dear Mr./Ms._____:

After careful consideration of the health department's application, we have decided not to concur with
that application. The application does not reflect our priorities for target populations or interventions
directed to those populations. Instead, the health department application proposes funding for programs
directed at the general public and a broadly targeted HIV counseling and testing program.
We do not make this decision lightly.

Our group spent many hours reviewing epidemiologic data and the results of our needs assessment to form
our population priorities. We also consulted with behavioral scientists and conducted an extensive literature
review to support our intervention priorities. The health department application appears not to have
recognized our efforts or recommendations.

We also want to register our dismay at the health department's lack of cooperation with the review
process. Initially the CPG was informed that we would have 24 hours to review the application and that
budget tables would not be included in the draft copy sent for review. We were able to negotiate three
days for the review, still an inadequate amount of time.

We would greatly appreciate your help in resolving this matter.

Sincerely,

Community Co-chair

APPENDIX C: Critical HIV Prevention Community Planning Attributes

The purpose of this section is to make explicit the critical attributes of the community planning objectives. These attributes were developed through a collaborative process that has included input from a variety of prevention partners including community and health department co-chairs, community planning technical assistance providers, the National Alliance of State and Territorial AIDS Directors, and CDC staff.

This Appendix groups attributes according to the objectives of community planning. If the designated attributes of an objective for a given jurisdiction are present in a community planning process, then one may with some level of confidence say that this objective is being met.

For evaluation purposes, designated indicators (Section VI: Accountability) have been explicitly developed based on these attributes. It is important to note that jurisdictions are not required to individually report on each attribute listed here. However, in the case of a letter of nonconcurrence, programmatic reviews conducted by CDC or a jurisdiction identified as having significant community planning challenges, the jurisdiction may be asked to provide evidence of applicable attributes.

> **OBJECTIVE A:** Implement an open recruitment process (outreach, nominations, and selection) for CPG membership. The presence of the following attributes are critical to achieving this Objective:

- ☐ **Attribute 1** *(Nominations)*: Presence of written procedures for nominations to the CPG.
- ☐ **Attribute 2** *(Nominations)*: Evidence that written procedures (above) were used for nominations to the CPG.
- ☐ **Attribute 3** *(Nominations)*: Evidence that a nominations committee has been established.
- ☐ **Attribute 4** *(Nominations)*: Evidence that nominations targeted membership gaps as identified by the community planning group.
- ☐ **Attribute 5** *(Selection)*: Evidence that membership decisions involve more than the health department staff.
- ☐ **Attribute 6** *(Selection)*: Written documentation of the process for selection of CPG members.
- ☐ **Attribute 7** *(Selection)*: Evidence that the process (above) was used in selection of CPG members.

OBJECTIVE B: Ensure that the CPG(s) membership is representative of the diversity of populations most at risk for HIV infection and community characteristics in the jurisdiction, and includes key professional expertise and representation from key governmental and non-governmental agencies. The presence of the following attributes are critical to achieving this Objective:

☐ **Attribute 8** *(Representation):* CPG includes: (a) members who represent populations most at risk for HIV infection as reflected in the current and projected epidemic, as documented in the prior year's epidemiologic profile, and (b) persons living with HIV/AIDS.

☐ **Attribute 9** *(Representation):* CPG membership includes members who represent the affected community in terms of race/ethnicity, gender/gender identity, sexual orientation, and geographic distribution.

☐ **Attribute 10** *(Representation):* CPG membership includes, or has access to, professional expertise in behavioral/social science, epidemiology, evaluation, and service provision.

☐ **Attribute 11** *(Representation):* CPG membership includes, or has access to, key government agencies, including: health department HIV/AIDS program and the state/local health department STD program staff.

☐ **Attribute 12** *(Representation):* CPG membership includes, or has access to, key governmental and non-governmental agencies with expertise in factors and issues relative to HIV prevention.

OBJECTIVE C: Foster a community planning process that encourages inclusion and parity among community planning members. The presence of the following attributes are critical to achieving this Objective:

☐ **Attribute 13** *(Inclusion):* Evidence of that to gain input from representatives of marginalized groups, who would be hard to recruit and/or retain as CPG members, the CPG convened ad hoc committees, panels, and/or focus groups.

☐ **Attribute 14** *(Inclusion):* Evidence that efforts were undertaken to accommodate or facilitate members who face challenging barriers (e.g., health care or economic needs) to their continued participation in the CPG.

☐ **Attribute 15** *(Inclusion):* Evidence of a clear decision-making process, including conflict of interest rules.

☐ **Attribute 16** *(Inclusion):* Evidence of an orientation, mentoring or training process for new CPG members.

☐ **Attribute 17** *(Inclusion):* Evidence that CPG meetings are open to the public and allow time for public comment.

☐ **Attribute 18** *(Parity):* Evidence of ongoing training process for all CPG members.

OBJECTIVE D: Carry out a logical, evidence-based process to determine the highest priority, population-specific prevention needs in the jurisdiction. The presence of the following attributes are critical to achieving this Objective:

☐ **Attribute 19** *(Epidemiologic Profile)*: The epidemiologic profile provides information about defined populations at high risk for HIV infection for the CPG to consider in the prioritization process.

☐ **Attribute 20** *(Epidemiologic Profile)*: Strengths and limitations of data sources used in the epidemiologic profile are described (general issues and jurisdiction-specific issues).

☐ **Attribute 21** *(Epidemiologic Profile)*: Data gaps are explicitly identified in the epidemiologic profile.

☐ **Attribute 22** *(Epidemiologic Profile)*: The epidemiologic profile contains a narrative interpretation of data presented.

☐ **Attribute 23** *(Epidemiologic Profile)*: Evidence that the epidemiologic profile was presented to the CPG members prior to the prioritization process.

☐ **Attribute 24** *(Community Services Assessment)*: The Community Services Assessment (CSA) focuses on one or more high priority populations (i.e., substantially contributing to new HIV infections in a jurisdiction) identified in the epidemiologic profile.

☐ **Attribute 25** *(Community Services Assessment)*: Data are gathered that define populations' needs in terms of knowledge, skills, attitudes, and norms.

☐ **Attribute 26** *(Community Services Assessment)*: Data are gathered that define populations' needs in terms of access to services.

☐ **Attribute 27** *(Community Services Assessment):* The CSA details the target populations being served.

☐ **Attribute 28** *(Community Services Assessment):* The CSA details the interventions provided to each target population.

☐ **Attribute 29** *(Community Services Assessment)*: The CSA describes the geographic coverage of interventions or programs.

☐ **Attribute 30** *(Community Services Assessment)*: The CSA was utilized in demonstrating linkages between the application and funded interventions.

☐ **Attribute 31** *(Community Services Assessment)*: Evidence that prior to the prioritization process, the CPG was provided with a summary of the CSA.

☐ **Attribute 32** *(Gap Analysis)*: The gap analysis includes data from the epidemiologic profile and CSA.

☐ **Attribute 33** *(Gap Analysis)*: A gap analysis specifically identifies both met and unmet needs.

☐ **Attribute 34** *(Gap Analysis)*: The gap analysis identifies the portion of needs being met with CDC funds.

☐ **Attribute 35** *(Gap Analysis)*: Evidence that prior to the prioritization process, the CPG was provided with a summary of the gap analysis findings.

☐ **Attribute 36** *(Gap Analysis)*: The gap analysis was utilized by the CPG in demonstrating linkages between the application and funded interventions

OBJECTIVE E: Ensure that priority target populations are based on an epidemiologic profile and a community services assessment. The presence of the following attributes are critical to achieving this Objective:

☐ **Attribute 37** *(Target Populations)*: Evidence that the size of at-risk populations was considered in setting priorities for target populations.

☐ **Attribute 38** *(Target Populations)*: Evidence that a measurement of the percentage of HIV morbidity (i.e., HIV/AIDS incidence or prevalence), if available, was considered in setting priorities for target populations.

☐ **Attribute 39** *(Target Populations)*: Evidence that the prevalence of risky behaviors in the population was considered in setting priorities for target populations.

☐ **Attribute 40** *(Target Populations)*: Target populations are defined by transmission risk, gender, age, race/ethnicity, HIV status, and geographic location.

☐ **Attribute 41** *(Target Populations)*: Target populations are rank ordered by priority, in terms of their contribution to new HIV infections.

OBJECTIVE F: Ensure that prevention activities/interventions for identified priority target populations are based on behavioral and social science, outcome effectiveness, and/or have been adequately tested with intended consumers for cultural appropriateness, relevance, and acceptability. The presence of the following attributes are critical to achieving this Objective:

☐ **Attribute 42** *(Prevention Activities/Interventions)*: Demonstrated application of existing behavioral and social science, and pre- and post-test outcome evidence (including evaluation date, when available) to show effectiveness in averting or reducing high-risk behavior within the target population.

☐ **Attribute 43** *(Prevention Activities/Interventions)*: Evidence that the prevention activity/intervention is acceptable to the target population (e.g., testing, focus groups, etc.).

☐ **Attribute 44** *(Prevention Activities/Interventions)*: Evidence that the prevention activity/intervention is feasible to implement for the intended population in the intended setting.

☐ **Attribute 45** *(Prevention Activities/Interventions)*: Evidence that the prevention activity/intervention was developed by or with input from the target population.

☐ **Attribute 46** *(Prevention Activities/Interventions)*: Prevention activities/interventions are characterized by focus, level, factors expected to affect risk, setting, and frequency/duration.

☐ **Attribute 47** *(Prevention Activities/Interventions)*: Each prevention activity/intervention is also characterized by scale and significance.

☐ **Attribute 48** *(Prevention Activities/Interventions)*: Prevention activities/interventions are prioritized by risk population and their ability to have the greatest impact on decreasing new infections.

Objective G: Demonstrate a direct relationship between the Comprehensive HIV Prevention Plan and the Health Department Application for federal HIV prevention funding. The presence of the following attributes are critical to achieving this Objective:

☐ **Attribute 49** *(Comprehensive Plan)*: Explicit demonstration of linkages between the comprehensive HIV prevention plan and the health department application to CDC for federal funding.

☐ **Attribute 50** *(Comprehensive Plan)*: Letter of Concurrence.

Objective H: Demonstrate a direct relationship between the Comprehensive HIV Prevention Plan and funded interventions. The presence of the following attributes are critical to achieving this Objective:

☐ **Attribute 51** *(Comprehensive Plan)*: Explicit demonstration of linkages between the comprehensive HIV prevention plan and funded interventions.

☐ **Attribute 52** *(Community Services Assessment)*: Explicit demonstration that the CPG has used the CSA to determine whether interventions were funded according to the comprehensive HIV prevention plan.

APPENDIX D: Glossary of HIV Prevention Terms

> Note: The definitions used here are specific to how the terms are used in CDC Program Announcement 04-012 and the HIV Prevention Community Planning Guidance

Accountability: An obligation or willingness to accept responsibility.

Application: A health department's formal request to CDC for HIV prevention funding. The application contains a written narrative and budget reflecting the priorities described in the jurisdiction's comprehensive HIV prevention plan.

Behavioral data: Information collected from studies that examine human behavior relevant to disease risk. For instance, relevant behavioral data for HIV risk may include sexual activity, substance use, condom use, etc.

Behavioral intervention: See "Intervention."

Capacity building: Activities that strengthen the core competencies of an organization and contribute to its ability to develop and implement an effective HIV prevention intervention and sustain the infrastructure and resource base necessary to support and maintain the intervention.

CARE Act: The Ryan White Comprehensive AIDS Resources Emergency (CARE) Act, the primary federal legislation created to address the health and support service needs of persons in the United States living with HIV/AIDS, and their families. Enacted in 1990, the CARE Act was re-authorized in 1996.

Centers for Disease Control and Prevention (CDC): The lead federal agency for protecting the health and safety of people, providing credible information to enhance health decisions, and promoting health through strong partnerships. Based in Atlanta, Georgia., this agency of the U.S. Department of Health and Human Services serves as the national focus for developing and applying disease prevention and control, environmental health, and health promotion and education activities designed to improve the health of the people of the United States.

Collaboration: Working with another person, organization, or group for mutual benefit by exchanging information, sharing resources, or enhancing the other's capacity, often to achieve a common goal or purpose.

Community-level intervention (CLI): An intervention that seeks to improve the risk conditions and behaviors in a community through a focus on the community as a whole, rather than by intervening only with individuals or small groups. This is often done by attempting to alter social norms, policies, or characteristics of the environment. Examples of CLI include community mobilizations, social marketing campaigns, community-wide events, policy interventions, and structural interventions.

Community planning group (CPG): The official HIV prevention planning body that follows the *HIV Prevention Community Planning Guidance* to develop a comprehensive HIV prevention plan for a project area.

Community services assessment: A description of the prevention needs of populations at risk for HIV infection, the prevention interventions/activities implemented to address these needs (regardless of funding source), and service gaps. The community services assessment is comprised of:

- RESOURCE INVENTORY - Current HIV prevention and related resources and activities in the project area, regardless of the funding source. A comprehensive resource inventory includes information regarding HIV prevention activities within the project area and other education and prevention activities that are likely to contribute to HIV risk reduction.
- NEEDS ASSESSMENT - A process for obtaining and analyzing information to determine the current status and service needs of a defined population or geographic area.
- GAP ANALYSIS - a description of the unmet HIV prevention needs within the high-risk populations defined in the epidemiologic profile. The unmet needs are identified by a comparison of the needs assessment and resource inventory.

Comprehensive HIV prevention plan: A plan that identifies prioritized target populations and describes what interventions will best meet the needs of each prioritized target population. The primary task of the community planning process is developing a comprehensive HIV prevention plan through a participatory, science-based planning process. The contents of the plan are described in the *HIV Prevention Community Planning Guidance*, and key information necessary to develop the comprehensive HIV prevention plan is found in the epidemiologic profile and the community services assessment.

Concurrence: The community planning group's (CPG's) agreement that the health department's application for HIV prevention funds reflects the CPG's target populations and intervention priorities (see "nonconcurrence"). As part of its application to the CDC for federal HIV prevention funds, every health department must include a letter of concurrence, concurrence with reservations or nonconcurrence from each CPG officially convened and recognized in the jurisdiction.

Conflict of interest: Conflict between the private interests and public obligations of a person in an official position.

Cooperative agreement: A financial assistance mechanism that may be used instead of a grant when the awarding office anticipates substantial federal programmatic involvement with the recipient.

Coordination: Aligning processes, services, or systems, to achieve increased efficiencies, benefits or improved outcomes. Examples of coordination may include sharing information, such as progress reports, with state and local health departments, or structuring prevention delivery systems to reduce duplication of effort.

Cost-effectiveness: The relative costs and effectiveness of proposed strategies and interventions, either demonstrated or probable.

Culturally appropriate: Conforming to a culture's acceptable expressions and standards of behavior and thoughts. Interventions and educational materials are more likely to be culturally appropriate when representatives of the intended target audience are involved in planning, developing, and pilot testing them.

Demographics: The statistical characteristics of human populations such as age, race, ethnicity, sex, and size.

Diversity: Individual differences along the dimensions of race, ethnicity, gender, sexual orientation, socio-economic status, age, physical abilities, religious beliefs, political beliefs, health or disease status, or other ideologies. The concept of diversity encompasses acceptance, respect, and understanding that each individual is unique.

Epidemic: The rapid spread, growth, or occurrence of cases of an illness, specific health-related behavior, or other health-related events in a community or region in excess of normal expectancy.

Epidemiologic profile: A document that describes the HIV/AIDS epidemic within various populations and identifies characteristics of both HIV-infected and HIV-negative persons in defined geographic areas. It is composed of information gathered to describe the effect of HIV/AIDS on an area in terms of sociodemographic, geographic, behavioral, and clinical characteristics. The epidemiologic profile serves as the scientific basis for the identification and prioritization of HIV prevention and care needs in any given jurisdiction.

Epidemiology: The study of the causes, spread, control and prevention of disease in human beings.

Evidenced-based: Behavioral, social, and structural interventions that are relevant to HIV risk reduction, have been tested using a methodologically rigorous design, and have been shown to be effective in a research setting. These evidence- or science-based interventions have been evaluated using behavioral or health outcomes; have been compared to a control/comparison group(s) (or pre-post data without a comparison group if a policy study); had no apparent bias when assigning persons to intervention or control groups or were adjusted for any apparent assignment bias; and, produced significantly greater positive results when compared to the control/comparison group(s), while not producing negative results.

CDC expects its grantees to deliver interventions based on a range of evidence. These interventions may include:

* Evidenced-based interventions (that meet the criteria described above and can be found in CDC's Compendium of HIV Prevention Interventions with Evidence of Effectiveness (1999). These interventions can either be implemented exactly as intended and within a context similar to the original intervention or adapted and tailored to a different target population if the core elements of the intervention are maintained.

* Interventions with insufficient evidence of effectiveness based on prior outcome monitoring data suggesting positive effects, but that cannot be rigorously proven. These interventions must be based on sound science and theory; a logic model that matches the science

and theory to the intended outcomes of interest; and a logic model that matches relevant behavioral-epi data from their community and target population.

Group-level interventions (GLIs): Health education and risk-reduction counseling that shifts the delivery of service from the individual to groups of varying sizes. Group-level interventions use peer and non-peer models involving a range of skills, information, education, and support.

Health communications/public information (HC/PI): The delivery of planned HIV/AIDS prevention messages through one or more channels to target audiences. The messages are designed to build general support for safe behavior, support personal risk-reduction efforts, and inform people at risk for infection about how to get specific services. Channels of delivery include electronic media, print media, hotlines, clearinghouses, and presentations/lectures.

Health education/risk reduction (HE/RR): Organized efforts to reach people at increased risk of becoming HIV-infected or, if already infected, of transmitting the virus to others. The goal is to reduce the spread of infection. Activities range from individual HIV prevention counseling to broad, community-based interventions.

High-risk behavior: A behavior in a high prevalence setting that places an individual at risk for HIV or STDs or in any setting in which either partner is infected.

HIV prevention community planning: The cyclical, evidence-based planning process in which authority for identifying priorities for funding HIV prevention programs is vested

in one or more planning groups in a state or local health department that receives HIV prevention funds from CDC.

HIV prevention counseling: An interactive process between client and counselor aimed at identifying concrete, acceptable, and appropriate ways to reduce risky sex and needle-sharing behaviors related to HIV acquisition (for HIV-uninfected clients) or transmission (for HIV-infected clients).

Incidence: The number of new cases in a defined population within a certain time period, often a year, that can be used to measure disease frequency. It is important to understand the difference between HIV incidence, which refers to new cases, and new HIV diagnosis, which does not reflect when a person was infected.

Incidence rate: The number of new cases in a specific area during a specific time period among those at risk of becoming cases in the same area and time period. The incidence rate provides a measure of the impact of illness relative to the size of the population. Incidence rate is calculated by dividing incidence in the specified period by the population in which cases occurred. A multiplier is used to convert the resulting fraction to a number over a common denominator, often 100,000.

Inclusion: Meaningful involvement of members in the process with an active voice in decision-making. An inclusive process assures that the views, perspectives, and needs of all affected communities are actively included.

Individual-level interventions (ILIs): Health education and risk-reduction counseling provided for one individual at a time. ILIs help clients make plans for behavior change and ongoing appraisals of their own behavior and include skills-building activities. These interventions also facilitate linkages to services in both clinic and community settings (for example, substance abuse treatment settings) in support of behaviors and practices that prevent transmission of HIV, and help clients make plans to obtain these services.

Injection drug user (IDU): Someone who uses a needle to inject drugs into his or her body.

Intervention: A specific activity (or set of related activities) intended to change the knowledge, attitudes, beliefs, behaviors, or practices of individuals and populations to reduce their health risk. An intervention has distinct process and outcome objectives and a protocol outlining the steps for implementation.

Intervention plan: A plan setting forth the goals, expectations, and implementation procedures for an intervention. It should describe the evidence or theory basis for the intervention, justification for application to the target population and setting, and the service delivery plan.

Jurisdiction: An area or region that is the responsibility of a particular governmental agency. This term usually refers to an area where a state or local health department monitors HIV prevention activities (e.g., Jonestown is within the jurisdiction of the Jones County Health Department).

Logic model: A systematic and visual way to present and share understanding of the relationships among the resources available to operate a program, planned activities, and anticipated changes or results. The most basic logic model is a picture of how a program will work. It uses words and/or pictures to describe the sequence of activities thought to bring about change and how these activities are linked to the results the program is expected to achieve.

Management and staffing plan: A plan describing the roles, responsibilities, and relationships of all staff in the program, regardless of funding source. An organization chart provides a visual description of these relationships.

Men who have sex with men (MSM): Men who report sexual contact with other men (that is, homosexual contact) and men who report sexual contact with both men and women (that is, bisexual contact), whether or not they identify as "gay."

Met need: A need within a specific target population for HIV prevention services that is currently being addressed through existing HIV prevention resources. These resources are available to, appropriate for, and accessible to that population (as determined through the community services assessment of prevention needs). For example, a project area with an organization for African American gay, bisexual, lesbian, and transgender individuals may meet the HIV/AIDS education needs of African American men who have sex with men through its outreach, public information, and group counseling efforts. An unmet need is a requirement for HIV prevention services within a specific target population that is not currently being addressed through existing HIV prevention services and activities, either because no services are available or because available services are either inappropriate for or inaccessible to the target population. For example, a project area lacking Spanish-language HIV counseling and testing services will not meet the needs of Latinos with limited-English proficiency.

MSM/IDU: Men who report both sexual contact with other men and injection drug use as risk factors for HIV infection.

Nonconcurrence: A Community Planning Group's disagreement with the program priorities identified in the health department's application for CDC funding. Nonconcurrence also may mean that a CPG has determined that the health department has not fully collaborated in developing the comprehensive plan.

Outcome evaluation: Evaluation employing rigorous methods to determine whether the prevention program has an effect on the predetermined set of goals. The use of such methods allows ruling out factors that might otherwise appear responsible for the changes seen. These measurements assess the effects of interventions on client outcomes such as knowledge, attitudes, beliefs, and behavior.

Outcome monitoring: Efforts to track the progress of clients or a program based upon outcome measures set forth in program goals. These measurements assess the effects of interventions on client outcomes such as knowledge, attitudes, beliefs, and behavior. Monitoring allows the identification of changes that occurred, but the intervention may not have been

responsible for the change. This would take a more rigorous approach (see Outcome evaluation).

Outreach: HIV/AIDS interventions generally conducted by peer or paraprofessional educators face-to-face with high-risk individuals in neighborhoods or other areas where they typically congregate. Outreach may include distribution of condoms and educational materials as well as HIV testing. A major purpose of outreach activities is to encourage those at high risk to learn their HIV status.

Parity: The ability of community planning group members to equally participate and carry-out planning tasks or duties in the community planning process. To achieve parity, representatives should be provided with opportunities for orientation and skills-building to participate in the planning process, and have equal voice in voting and other decision-making activities.

Partner counseling and referral services (PCRS): A systematic approach to notifying sex and needle-sharing partners of HIV-infected persons of their possible exposure to HIV so they can avoid infection or, if already infected, prevent transmission to others. PCRS helps partners gain earlier access to individualized counseling, HIV testing, medical evaluation, treatment, and other prevention services.

PLWHA: A person or persons living with HIV or AIDS.

Prevalence: The total number of cases of a disease in a given population at a particular point in time. For HIV/AIDS surveillance, prevalence refers to living persons with HIV disease, regardless of time of infection or diagnosis date. Prevalence does not give an indication of how long a person has had a disease and cannot be used to calculate rates of disease. It can provide an estimate of risk that an individual will have a disease at a point in time.

Prevention activity: Activity that focuses on behavioral interventions, structural interventions, capacity building, or information gathering.

Prevention case management (PCM): Client-centered HIV prevention activity with the fundamental goal of promoting the adoption of HIV risk-reduction behaviors by clients with multiple, complex problems and risk-reduction needs. PCM is a hybrid of HIV risk-reduction counseling and traditional case management, which provide intensive, ongoing, and individualized prevention counseling, support, and service brokerage.

Prevalence rate: The number of people living with a disease or condition in a defined population on a specified date, divided by that population. It is often expressed per 100,000 persons.

Prevention need: A documented necessity for HIV prevention services within a specific target population. The documentation is based on numbers, proportions, or other estimates of the impact of HIV or AIDS among this population from the epidemiologic profile. Prevention need also is based on information from the epidemiologic profile and community services assessment.

Prevention program: An organized effort to design and implement one or more

interventions to achieve a set of predetermined goals, for example, to increase condom use with non-steady partners.

Prevention services: Interventions, strategies, programs, and structures designed to change behavior that may lead to HIV infection or other diseases. Examples of HIV prevention services include street outreach, educational sessions, condom distribution, and mentoring and counseling programs.

Priority set of prevention interventions/ activities: A set of interventions/activities identified in the Comprehensive HIV Prevention Plan, which, if implemented, can have a major effect on the HIV epidemic in a target population.

Priority population: A population identified through the epidemiologic profile and community services assessment that requires prevention efforts due to high rates of HIV infection and the presence of risky behavior.

Program announcement: A CDC announcement in the Federal Register describing the amount of funding available for a particular public health goal and soliciting applications for funding. The program announcement describes required activities and asks the applicants to describe how they will carry out the required activities.

Program indicator: A quantitative measure of program performance.

Public information program: Activities funded through the cooperative agreement to build general support for safe behavior, dispel myths about HIV/AIDS, address barriers to effective risk reduction programs, and support efforts for personal risk reduction. In addition to addressing general audiences, public information programs should inform persons at risk of infection about how to obtain specific prevention and treatment services such as counseling, testing, referral, partner counseling and referral services, and STD screening and treatment.

Project area: Same as "Jurisdiction."

Qualitative data: Non-numeric data, including information from sources such as narrative behavior studies, focus group interviews, open-ended interviews, direct observations, ethnographic studies, and documents. Findings from these sources are usually described in terms of underlying meanings, common themes, and patterns of relationships rather than numeric or statistical analysis. Qualitative data often complement and help explain quantitative data.

Quantitative data: Numeric information — such as numbers, rates, and percentages — representing counts or measurements suitable for statistical analysis.

Referral: A process by which immediate client needs for prevention, care, and supportive services are assessed and prioritized and clients are provided with assistance in identifying and accessing services (such as, setting up appointments and providing transportation). Referral does not include ongoing support or case management. There should be a strong working relationship with other providers and agencies that might be able to provide needed services.

Relevance: The extent to which an intervention plan addresses the needs of affected populations in the jurisdiction and other community stakeholders. As described in the *Guidance*, relevance is the extent to which the populations targeted in the intervention plan are consistent with the target populations in the comprehensive HIV prevention plan.

Representation: The act of serving as an official member reflecting the perspective of a specific community. A representative should reflect that community's values, norms, and behaviors, and have expertise in understanding and addressing the specific HIV prevention needs of the population. Representatives also must be able to participate in the group and objectively weigh the overall priority prevention needs of the jurisdiction.

Representative: A sample having the same distribution of characteristics as the population from which it is drawn. Thus the sample can be used to draw conclusions about the population.

Risk factor or risk behavior: Behavior or other factor that places a person at risk for disease. For example, drug use is a factor that increases risk of acquiring HIV infection; and factors such as sharing injection drug use equipment, unprotected anal or vaginal sexual contact, and commercial unprotected sex increase the risk of acquiring and transmitting HIV.

Seroprevalence: The number of people in a population who test HIV-positive based on serology (blood serum) specimens. Seroprevalence is often presented as a percent of the total specimens tested or as a rate per 1,000 persons tested.

Science-based: See "Evidence-based."

Sociodemographic factors: Important background information about the population of interest, such as age, sex, race, educational status, income, and geographic location. These factors are often thought of as explanatory, because they help make sense of the results of analyses.

Socioeconomic status (SES): A description of a person's societal status using factors or measurements such as income levels, relationship to the national poverty line, educational achievement, neighborhood of residence, or home ownership.

Structural intervention: An intervention designed to implement or change laws, policies, physical structures, social or organizational structures, or standard operating procedures to affect environmental or societal change. (An example might be changing the operating hours of a testing site or providing bus tokens for access.)

Surveillance: The ongoing and systematic collection, analysis, and interpretation of data about occurrences of a disease or health condition.

Target populations: Populations that are the focus of HIV prevention efforts because they have high rates of HIV infection and high levels of risky behavior. Groups are often identified using a combination of behavioral risk factors and demographic characteristics.

Technical assistance (TA): The delivery of expert programmatic, scientific, and technical support to organizations and communities in the design, implementation, evaluation of HIV prevention interventions and programs. CDC funds a National Technical Assistance Providers' Network to assist HIV prevention community planning groups in all phases of the community planning process.

Transmission categories: Classification of infected individuals based on how the individual may have been exposed to HIV, such as injection drug use.

Unmet need: See "Met need."

Printed in Great Britain
by Amazon

ISBN 9781499572124

90000

9 781499 572124

THE CAVE OF SANTA CLOPS

BY GIG WAILGUM